How to manage Dry Eyes sustainably

By Shiv Kumar

Disclaimer

The information provided in this book is intended for informational and educational purposes only. It is not a substitute for professional medical advice, diagnosis, or treatment.

For your individual requirements, you should consult an ophthalmologist or a corresponding medical professional.

Contents

Preface

In the wake of increasing modernization, humans have found solutions to many of life's problems. However, this same modernization has also given rise to several new challenges that were either less prominent or non-existent in the past.

One such issue is Dry Eyes. Whether you call it an issue or a disease, it remains a significant problem that an increasing number of people are grappling with today. Dry Eyes is not confined to a specific country or region; it is a global concern. Despite its widespread prevalence, it doesn't garner as much attention as life-threatening diseases like cancer or heart attacks. And the reason is simple: it doesn't pose a direct threat to life.

However, it does impact the quality of life, and there's no reason why one should compromise on that. Those suffering from Dry Eyes can attest to the impact it has on their daily lives.

Many of you might have already invested a considerable amount of money in laser treatments, consultations with ophthalmologists, and a plethora of eye drops. These treatments are not futile; they do provide some relief. But the question remains, 'Are these solutions sustainable?' If your answer is 'no,' then this book is for you.

In this book, I will delve into the root causes of this problem and guide you on how to reduce your dependence on numerous eye drops, tablets, and frequent visits to the ophthalmologist.

How do you know if you are suffering from Dry Eyes?

It can take a long time for you to realize that the constant discomfort and uneasiness in your eyes are not due to other factors, but dry eyes.

People with vision issues often attribute this discomfort to their eyeglasses.

So, if you are seeing any of the symptoms like below, do check if you are suffering from dry eyes:

1. Decreased tear production
2. Constant itching and discomfort in the eyes
3. A persistent feeling of uneasiness in the eyes
4. Reduced frequency of automatic blinking
5. A sensation of a foreign particle in the eyes

In order to confirm that you have a dry eyes issue, you do need to visit an ophthalmologist.

Schirmer's test (paper in the eye test) and Tear break-up time using an ophthalmic instrument are some of the ways in which issue of dry eyes can be confirmed.

What happens to your eyes in Dry Eyes?

In a completely healthy eye, there is a continuous presence of a tear layer. Tears play a crucial role in maintaining eye health by keeping it lubricated, transporting vital nutrients, fighting infections, and removing foreign impurities.

Tears are composed of three substances – water, oil, and mucus. Any imbalance in their proportions or quality can impact the quantity or quality of tears, leading to dry eyes.

During dry eyes, there is an insufficient presence of tears on the cornea. Once the tear film is absent, your body registers this event and attempts to combat it, leading to inflammation. Interestingly, inflammation can also trigger the absence of the tear film. Thus, inflammation leads to dry eyes, and dry eyes further lead to inflammation, creating a vicious cycle. And I will tell you what you need to do to exit this viscous cycle. But you need to wait a little for that as I will first provide the details on the effects of Dry Eyes and the traditional solutions for it.

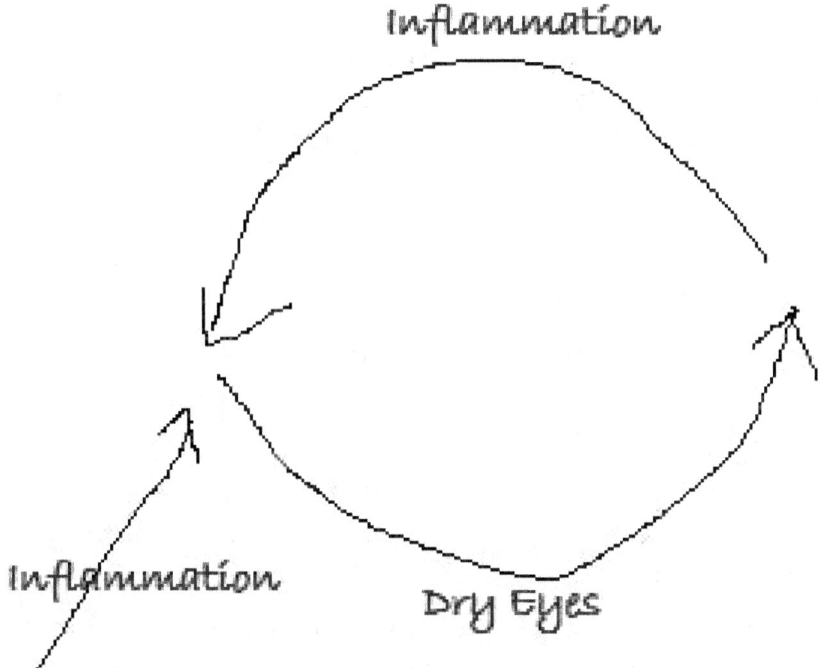

Inflammation
Inflammation
Dry Eyes

Issues you face due to Dry Eyes

If dry eyes were a condition where only your eyes are a little dry and rest of your body functions are completely unscathed, you might not have had difficulties managing it. However, that is not the case. The workings of your eyes are very much connected to the functions of other parts of your body. Put it simply, it will affect other parts of your body, the quality of your life, and a lot of other things around it. Some of it are listed below.

<u>Restlessness</u>: As the inflammation increases and the dryness in the eyes also goes up, you will start to feel restless until you take an artificial tear or some other remedy.

<u>Uneasiness</u>: This is also similar to restlessness, where though your vision will not be hampered but you will have a feeling that some issue exists in your eyes.

<u>Stress</u>: Since you cannot keep taking eye drops every 10 minutes, your eyes will continuously ask for a lubrication. Till the time the tear gets up on the cornea, a tension will build and keep increasing your stress levels.

<u>Cortisol</u>: The increase in stress will cause the cortisol in your body to increase. For those who do not know what is cortisol, it is a hormone released by your body to fight stress.

<u>Decrease in Energy Levels</u>: This is completely expected as the energy in your body is spent fighting the stress. You will have less energy for your work.

<u>Changes in mood</u>: With all the things covered above, your mood is going to be definitely impacted. This can affect both your personal and work life.

Do you see now, how this all can affect you? This is how it can decrease your overall quality of your life.

Typical Solutions in the market

Below are some of the typical solutions that you will be provided or suggested by an ophthalmologist.

Artificial Tear Drops: This will be given to you to lubricate your eyes. You might be asked to take it frequently throughout the day. It is like an artificial replacement for the tears in your eyes.

Cyclosporin: Cyclosporin is a potent immunosuppressive drug that works by inhibiting T cell activation, thereby reducing the body's immune response. Generally, ophthalmologist suggest taking it for not more than a couple of years.

Steroids: A much stronger eye drop than the cyclosporin, steroids can help in some dry eyes' problems quickly. However, it is not at all suggested to use it for a long time due to potential side effects.

Laser Techniques: This is a more recent advancement where some laser technologies are used to selectively destroy blood vessels and use this to improve the function of the meibomian glands.

Warm Compresses: You may also be recommended a warm compress near your eyes to help better expression of meibum from the corresponding glands.

Gel or ointment: You may also be asked to apply a gel or similar liquid in your eyes.

Although the above solutions give you some benefits, they are unlikely to be sustainable.

Why are Traditional approaches not sustainable?

Most *artificial tear drops* contains preservatives. And your eyes will not like it if you take it for a long time.

Cyclosporin is an immunosuppressant and you are not recommended to take this all your life.

Steroids are strong medicines, and they can have side effects. As such, you can use it just at instances for few days. You cannot depend much on it for long term.

Laser Techniques are the costliest of all the traditional approaches discussed. Additionally, you would generally be required to undergo multiple laser sessions. And will that get rid of dry eyes problem forever? Likely not! It gives relief for a few months. And then you will most likely need more laser sessions, drilling a big hole in your pocket.

Warm compresses are a good habit you can inculcate and it can help a little. In fact, out of all the traditional methods, this can be sustainable but you may not get much benefit from it if you are having dry eyes problem for a long time.

The *gel and ointment* also are also an additional expense with not much promise to provide substantial relief.

And the main reason why these solutions don't provide sustainable results is because most of them work on reducing and alleviating the symptoms. Some also work on reducing inflammation. But then why is there an inflammation?

What is the root cause of Dry Eyes?

Many may believe that inflammation is the root cause of dry eyes. I don't agree with this completely. Because though it is a cause of dry eye, it is not the root cause. Since, the inflammation itself is caused by yet another source, which causes the inflammation. Hence, to treat dry eyes effectively, you need to manage the cause of inflammation.

The most likely cause of inflammation would be your lifestyle and/or lack of any key nutrients in the body.

Have you looked at the composition of the food that you eat? Well, some people can get away with eating just about anything. But not all can do that.

Television, Computer, Laptop, Mobile, and Tab are the inventions of the modern world. They have offered a lot of benefits to this world. But does your eye enjoy looking at the screen for 12 hrs daily? I guess not. And then there is a growing trend of screen interactions at night.

Water is available in plenty on this planet. A large percentage of your body is just water, which people lose through various channels throughout the day. Don't you think you need to make amends for what is getting lost?

Chairs, Table, and Sofas are fed up of holding your weight for so long day after day. They ask you to get up and be active. But you do not listen. Well, they will still be there for you. But don't overuse them so much.

Humans are social animal. Yet, some people don't prefer to socialize even the slightest. Everyone has their preferences, and you don't benefit from socializing complete day. But it does give benefits if you form a few good connections.

In some cases, your environmental conditions like temperature, humidity, air quality, and similar can also cause dry eye.

Sustainable Solutions for Dry Eyes

This is the most important chapter in this book. Though there is no guarantee, there are high chances that the methods and approaches that follow can yield better and more sustainable results to decrease your dry eyes problems.

Sun: The source of everything on this planet is our star 'Sun.' Without it there will be no life. And in the rawest form, this is what drives all life on earth. Even animals can be observed basking in the early morning sunlight. It is the primary and biggest source of vitamin D for your body. Perhaps the only source for vegetarians. Apart from that, it seems that the universe was designed to get a lot more from our sun. That's where the seasons on this planet changes every few months.

The sun's heat can work wonders on your body. So, go out for 10-15 minutes to bask in the warm sun rays during sunrise and the sunset.

Boiled Egg: If there is one item which I truly found to be a super food, it is egg. It also solves the problem of vitamin D for regions where there is not sufficient sunlight. I know, it cannot replace sun and its benefits. But when you do not have an option, use what's best available to you. And it is not just vitamin D! There are plenty of other nutritional value to it in the form of other vitamins, minerals, energy, high quality protein, and more.

Mixed Dry Fruits: Dry fruits can be seen as a source of good nutrients in almost all articles for vitamins, minerals, and proteins. So, why not include it daily in your diet? And for the best results, you can take a mix of different dry fruits so that you get a bit of all the nutrients. Here you should also make it a point to soak certain dry fruits like 'almonds' in water and then peel off the skin before consuming them for favourable outcomes.

And make it a point to add enough of walnuts and/or chia seeds in your plate too. This can be very helpful for your dry eyes.

Balanced Diet: You can consume all the dry fruits in the world, but they cannot be a substitute of a balanced diet. So, make sure to include a lot of fruits and vegetables in your diet.

Further, eating at a proper time is also essential for keeping your body functioning efficiently at all times.

Reduce Sugar: Everyone knows this one. But it is difficult not to have sugar. What you can do here is replace the processed sugar with natural sugars like jaggery powder, honey, and similar.

There are a lot of soft drinks which contains plenty of sugar. They may taste good. But in long run there is not much value passed to your body in having it.

This is another reason why fruits become must in your diet as it also provides you with natural sugars. These replacements would help reduce sudden spikes in sugar levels in your blood.

Reduce refined wheat flour: Ideally, you should do away with refined wheat flour as it is very difficult for your body to process it.

Water Consumption: Your body contains approximately 60% water and your brain is composed of nearly 73% water. So, consume at least around 3 litre of water per day depending on various factors like your age, gender, work profile etc

Yoga: A lot of people think of yoga as just a set of poses. And many people stop practicing it just after a few sessions. But if you talk to people who have been doing it on a regular basis, you will get to know the many benefits that they have received from it. However, you should do this early in the morning for the best results.

Meditation: Just like yoga, meditation also helps to maintain fitness of your complete being. It helps you to decrease the stress. Complement it with yoga and your stress levels should go down even faster.

Mudras: Mudras are gestures or seal used in yoga. You can consider it as part of yoga only. They channel the flow of various life forces in your body. It can really help in balancing various elements in your body.

Exercise: Being physically active is really important in today's time. You can go to a gym; and do cardio or light weight exercises. Basic stretching also helps. And outdoor walking, jogging, and running are also great. All of these will strengthen your body. But avoid too much strain if your body does not like it.

Swimming: It is a low impact sport that exercises your full body. It is also gives you a rejuvenating experience and a lot of people feel refreshed after just 30 minutes of swimming. It is one of the best exercises for all age groups.

Hard stop on screen usage: When you continuously use the screen, the rate of your eye blink reduces. This does not give enough opportunity to your eyes to get lubricated. And night time usage of screens is worse. So, decide a time when you want to stop using screens at night. Additionally, whenever you use screens, take regular breaks in between to give your eyes some time to relax and lubricate itself.

To make this easier, you can also download a free tool called EyeRest20 or EyeRest30, which blacks out your screen for 60 seconds after every 20 or 30 minutes respectively. This should give your eyes the much needed rest while working continuously on laptop/computer screens.

Link for the tool:

https://github.com/shivkumar3020/eyerest30

https://github.com/shivkumar3020/eyerest20

Consume Warm Food: When you eat cold food, the heat required to burn the food would be taken from your body. It does no good to your body. So, try to consume warm food.

Leisure and Hobbies: Let's admit it. Work takes up a large chunk of life when you are awake. But it also adds to a bit of stress and sometime a lot. Indulging in leisure activities and hobbies like music, sports, gardening etc automatically uplifts your mood and your stress level gets managed better.

Socialize: A good walk down the road with a friend or a nice family vacation keeps you energized and lifts your mood.

So, spend time with your family and/or friends. You may also engage in a community work that contributes to something that you believe in. Overall, form a few connections and bond with a few people. Some people find animals to be great friends. This is also an excellent idea.

Work: We went through a lot of things that are not 'work.' But being active does not just means hitting the gym and exercising. You also need to work. Even if you have a lot of money, there is still a lot of things you can do.

Ayurveda: Ayurveda is also called the science of life. It focuses on balancing the different elements in the body. You may try the offering of ayurveda to balance various elements in your body and you should see some benefits.

Consume Oil and Ghee: Oil and Ghee are natural lubricants. You cannot do without it in your food. So, use it properly to your advantages by adding a little of high-quality oil and ghee.

A type of ayurvedic ghee called as triphala ghrit can work wonders for your body and eyes.

Castor Oil: This is one specific oil that can relax your eyes. But you do not need to consume it for that. You need to apply it over your eye lids overnight and then wash it the next morning.

Body Posture: People tend to neglect their postures while sitting or standing. It does no good to you. Start practising a good posture and see the benefits yourself.

Preservative free lubricant: If you need to lubricate your eyes using drops, a preservative free lubricant will make your eyes feel much more comfortable. So, try this variant.

Fresh Air: We talked about water earlier. Similarly, air is also a very vital component for your body. And I mean fresh air. Take fresh air of the early morning to feed your mind and body some pure oxygen.

Remove toxins from body: Lean is the new fashion. Remove toxins from your body. And see how fresh and energetic you feel. This helps your complete body.

Oiling the body: Regular oiling the body and scalp also helps.

For oiling hair, an easy way to do it would be to oil it in the night and wash it the next morning while bathing. This gives you the benefit of oil without any sticky feeling during the day time.

Wake up early: You can do a lot of changes to your life, but if you are waking up at 10 am in the morning, your lifestyle cannot be called good in any way.

Read food labels before consumption: You read about sugar and refined wheat flour in the earlier pages. But the problem is you do not know what a pack of biscuit contains except that it tastes sweet or salty. Read the nutritional label next time. The components are listed with decreasing order of their percentage in the product.

Actually, if you can do away with packaged foods, that would be even better.

Palm massage: Using your palm to massage around your eyes also helps in reducing fatigue of your eyes and helps it to function better.

Warm Milk with saffron: Saffron contains antioxidants, anti-inflammatory, and neuroprotective properties, which may also improve eye health.

Coffee (with jaggery powder): Coffee can bring a lot of benefits to your overall health. However, replace the sugar with a good substitute like jaggery powder and then consume it. Another option is to consume black coffee.

Here, please note that coffee is a diuretic, which can cause loss of water from your body. So, consume it based on your individual comfort.

Head and Body Massage: An occasional massage for your head and body can be exceptionally good. Massage will help to increase the blood flow to various parts of your body, thereby improve its functioning. And your stress levels will decrease too.

Probiotics: Your gut is like the core of your body. If your gut is not healthy, you can have excessive gas and indigestion. This can also contribute to issues in your body and your eyes.

So, you can add probiotics like curd or buttermilk to your diet. They provide good bacteria to keep your gut happy.

Direct Air-Conditioning: AC is also known to aggravate the dry eye issues. So, it is best to keep minimum exposure to air-conditioning, especially the direct exposure to your head.

Humidity: If the place that you live in or are surrounded by for most of your time lacks sufficient humidity, it can also affect your occular health and cause dry eye . So, check for the humidity level near your place and see if you can do anything to be in a place with more moisture.

Some people have benefited from a humidifier. You can also try it, if humidity is a concern at your place.

Positivity: Your mental health is also important to maintain your eye and overall health. So be positive and keep hope that your eye health will eventually improve.

Rise in Brahma Muhurta: There is a magical time period that starts 1hr 36 mins prior to sunrise and lasts for 48 mins. Rising in this period helps your body's and mind's function to sync with the natural cycles helping your entire system to become healthy once again.

You can take help of apps like SerenRise (Brahma Muhruta Time & Widget) to easily track brahma muhurta time for your location.

From the list of items discussed above, see what helps you most and use it. You do not need to use all the items listed above to get the results.

However, all the above solutions will contribute in small percentages in relieving you from the dry eye problems. When added together, you can see even better results.

Like the traditional solutions, the approach discussed above will also need its regular inculcation in your life. But these are more sustainable and will not cost you an arm and a leg.

A few may also need to use traditional approaches like typical eyedrops, ointments, IPL, and others to decrease the acuteness of dry eyes initially and then gradually progress towards the sustainable approaches.

So, use the details provided here judiciously based on your own requirements and comfort.

FAQs

1. There are so many mudras. Which are the mudras that I can use specifically for the eye health?

Ans. You should not restrict yourself to just a couple of mudras. Since, different mudra provide different benefits that can help you in varied ways.

However, you can still take a look at Prana mudra, Vayu mudra, Apan Vayu mudra, Varun mudra, Rudra mudra, Prtihvi mudra, and Ksepana mudra to name a few.

2. Which are the exercises that I can do regularly?

Ans. I can suggest marching, standing leg raise, and jumping jack.

3. Why is Egg suggested in the food?

Ans. Egg is a super food. Your body needs essential nutrients, vitamins, minerals, protein, and fat for the regular function. A lot of people miss out on key ingredients in their diet due to their food choices or other reasons. In such a situation, Egg can be a great food for your body.

4. I like refined wheat flour. Can I consume it a little?

Ans. It is your choice as to what you want to eat. But as a personal suggestion, I will suggest you to completely avoid it.

Refined wheat flour is the stuff that remains when the whole wheat is refined to remove the skin and the husk from the grain, thereby destroying the grain's nutritional content.

So, what remains after the refining is just calories. You may like the taste, but your body will not thank you for it.

5. I have heard about MGD(Meibomian Gland Dysfunction). Can you tell me more about it?

Ans. MGD or Meibomian Gland Dysfunction can be one of the causes of dry eye. Basically, the meibomian gland secretes the oil which forms one of the constituents of your tear. For a healthy and stable tear, proper quantity and quality of this oil is essential.

So, if your oil glands are not functioning properly, it can cause dry eye issue.

However, here too, MGD may itself be caused by some other issue, which can be the root cause of your dry eye issue.

6. Yoga is just a set of poses. How can yoga help me in dry eye?

Ans. A lot of people do make this mistake in considering yoga as just a set of poses. But, it is a lot more than that.

It works on your nervous system, massages your glands, strengthens your core, and helps your body in many more ways that you may not know.

7. And what about mudras. They are just gestures?

Ans. For a person looking from outside, they are just gestures. But when you look deeply, it can have far reaching effect on your body.

Basically, your body is a type of electrical system. Yes, there is a small electricity that flows in your body.

So, when you use specific gestures, certain circuits in the body are closed and loops are formed, which aids in flow of energy and electricity through different parts of your body in a particular way. This can really help the various parts of your body to function efficiently and restoring good health.

8. Why are dry fruits important in the diet?

Ans. At a fundamental level, dry fruits are fruits minus their water content. So, when the liquid or water are drained out, what remains is purely their nutritional content. So, when you eat dry fruits, you are consuming only high quality nutrients and hardly any junk.

And when you are eating mix dry fruits, you are taking in the best from each one of them.

For dry eyes in particular, walnuts can be great, as it contains omega-3 fatty acids, which plays a major role in the proper functioning of eyes.

Other sources of omega-3 fatty acids are chia seeds, flax seeds, and various types of fishes. Also, to provide your body the necessary amount of this nutrient, you need to also take adequate intake of the corresponding food item.

9. Can I consume ayurvedic medicines by myself?

Ans. It is not suggested to consume any medicine of any form before consulting with a corresponding practitioner. So, consult with one of the doctors and then you can take the medicine.

10. Should I join a gym to learn physical exercises?

Ans. Though it is not mandatory to join a gym to learn the basic physical exercises, you can still join a good gym to learn some of the exercises.

Once you learn them, you can then practice it on your own.

11. Which are the main glands involved in the tear system?

Ans. Mainly, there are two glands involved in the tear system. First is the lacrimal gland, which secretes the watery substance. Second is the meibomian gland, which provides the oil in your tears.

The mucus is provided by the conjunctiva.

Also, please note that the functions of your body are intercon-nected. So, these glands do not operate completely independently.

12. What are the other things I can do to lessen the impact of screen usage on my eyes?

Ans. You can turn on the night light or any similar feature in your device to cut the blue light from the screen.

You can also try reducing the brightness and color of the display.

Additionally, you should make it a point to not use the screen in a dark background.

13. Can you provide names of any more probiotic food items apart from curd and curd products?

Ans. Kimchi and Sauerkraut are alternative probiotic food items, which you can try.

14. Can I apply eye cosmetics?

Ans. Eye cosmetics are not recommended for people suffering from dry eye problems. Cosmetics contains chemicals and can prove unhealthy for your eyes. Due to possible toxicity, irritation, and allergy, it is not good for your occular health.

15. I have undergone LASIK or similar eye procedure. Is it possible to have dry eye after this?

Ans. Yes, a good percentage of people do experience some level of dryness in their eyes post the procedure. You should consult with your ophthalmologist for the issue.

16. Which vitamin intakes can aid to improve my eye health?

Ans. Ideally, you should consume a balanced diet that provides your body with all vitamins and minerals. However, for your occular health in particular, vitamins A, B_{12}, C, and D can be highly beneficial.

17. I have diabetes and kidney disease. Can these diseases cause dry eyes?

Ans. Yes, diabetes and kidney disease can also negatively impact your occular health and cause dry eyes. So, you should try to manage your sugar levels and also keep your kidneys healthy.

18. Can I use contact lenses?

Ans. Although, short term use of contact lenses may not pose any problems. Long term use can cause issues.

The way you use them also makes the difference.

If at all you need to use lenses, you should use daily disposable lenses.

19. What are the sources of dry eye issue?

Ans. The source can be categorized into three types.

1. External inflammatory factors.

2. Eyelid related factors - meibomian gland dysfunction and Blepharitis.

3. Nerve induced.

For a particular person, the source can be a single or a mix of the above 3 types.

And these sources of dry eye may itself be caused by other factors, which would form the root causes of dry eye.

20. Are there any other sustainable solutions that is not listed?

Ans. There can be a few. But majority of the sustainable solutions are already covered in this book.

Manuka Honey is another item which is known to reduce the issue of dry eye in some people.

However, you should check more details about it and consult with your ophthalmologist before using it.

21. How effective is IPL for dry eye?

Ans. IPL may help you get relief from dry eye. It helps in reducing the inflammation and unclogging the meibomian glands. But it is costly and its effect may not last very long. So, you can leverage IPL once to get some relief from dry eyes. And then you can work to avoid the root causes of your dry eye.

Before opting for IPL, you should consult with your ophthalmologist.

22. Is IPL procedure safe?

Ans. Generally, there shouldn't be a concern for undergoing an IPL procedure as your eyes are covered during the session. However, it is not recommended for people with certain skin conditions.

Please talk to your ophthalmologist to know more about IPL and its safety.

23. Can sjogren's syndrome cause dry eye?

Ans. Yes, sjogren's syndrome, in which the immune system mistakenly attacks the healthy cells, organs, and tissues of the body can also cause dry eye.

24. How can I get relief from dry eye caused by sjogren's syndrome?

Ans. The sustainable solutions for dry eye provided in this book should also help you to get relief from dry eye caused by sjogren's syndrome.

Yoga and related practices, lifestyle improvement, healthy diet, and exercise can strengthen your immune system and decrease inflammation, thereby helping you to get relief from dry eye caused by sjogren's syndrome.

You may not see the benefits immediately but gradually over time you should definitely see positive changes in your health.

25. Can you suggest some foods that have high anti-inflammatory properties?

Ans. Some of the most anti-inflammatory foods are berries, broccoli, avocados, green tea, peppers, mushrooms, grapes, turmeric, extra virgin olive oil, dark chocolate, cocoa, cherries, tomatoes, and saffron.

26. Should I consume the packaged curd purchased from the store?

Ans. I do no recommend using the packaged curd due to the possibility of preservatives and also the staleness.

If you can set the curd at your home, that would be much better. Also, try to consume the curd soon after it has set, as later the curd can go sour and may not provide the best of benefits.

27. Are there any other ways to feel relaxed when feeling stressed or uneasy?

Ans. You can also try to activate your vagus nerve which can lead you to a state of feeling more relaxed and calm.

In order to do that, sit on a chair with a straight back, and hands on your thighs.

Breathe in deeply for 6 counts, then hold the breath for a count of 4. Next breathe out for a count of 8 and then hold that position for 6 counts.

Repeat the cycle for 5-10 minutes and you should experience calmness and relaxation.

You can also do this exercise in Sukhasana pose.

I hope this book was useful in helping you better understand your problems related to dry eyes. And most importantly the ways in which you can work to manage it more sustainably.

If you liked this book and it helped you in anyway, do share it with anyone in your family or friends, who can benefit from it.

You may also share a review about what you liked in the book.

Wishing everyone a healthy life.

Other Books Of Shiv Kumar

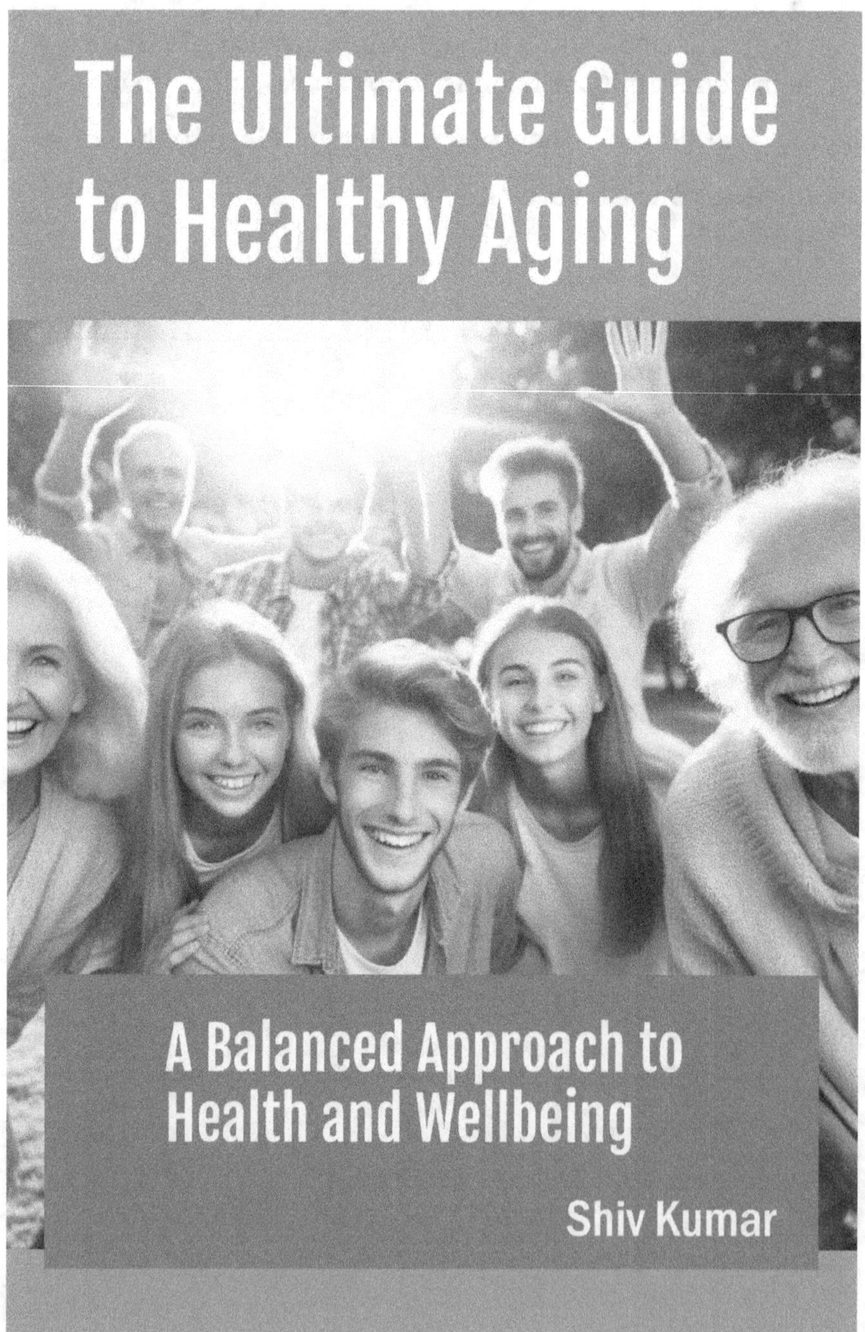

Other Books For You To Read

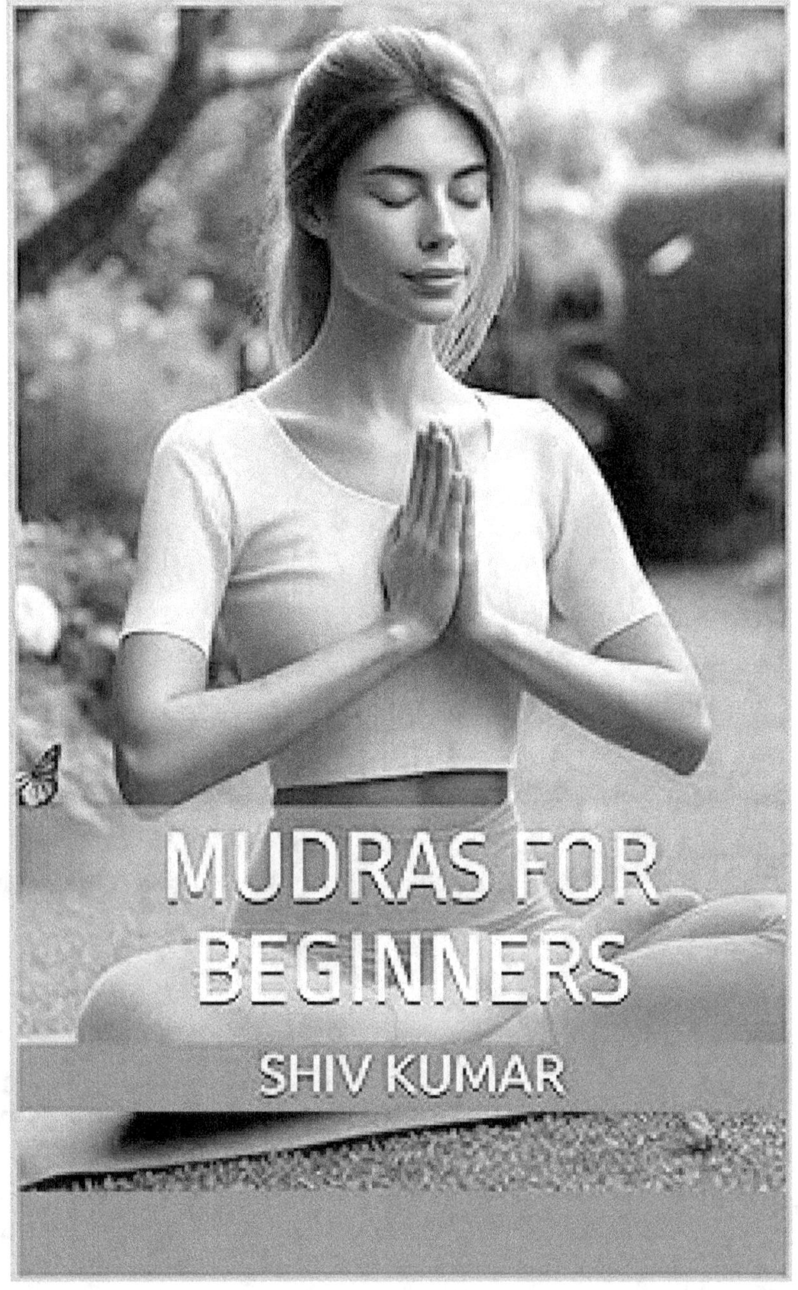

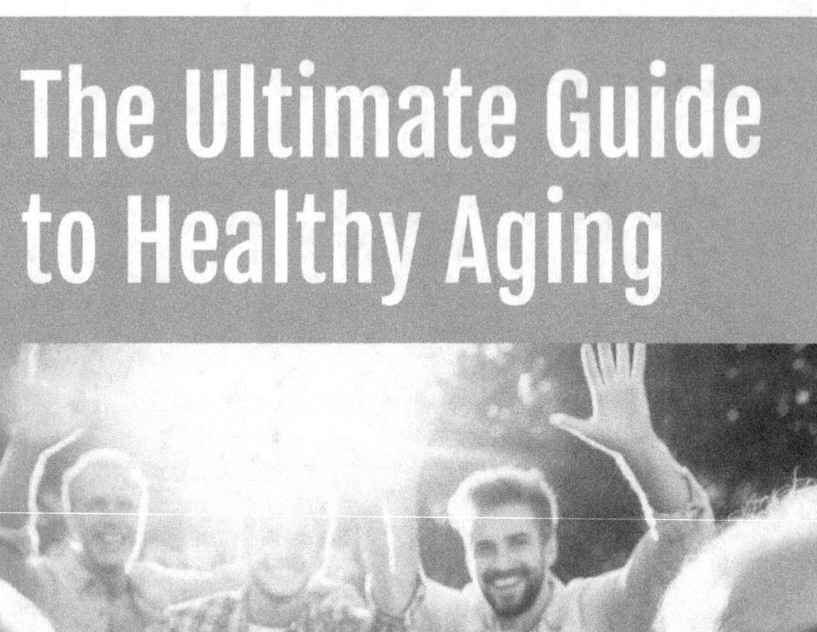
The Ultimate Guide
to Healthy Aging
A Balanced Approach to
Health and Wellbeing
Shiv Kumar

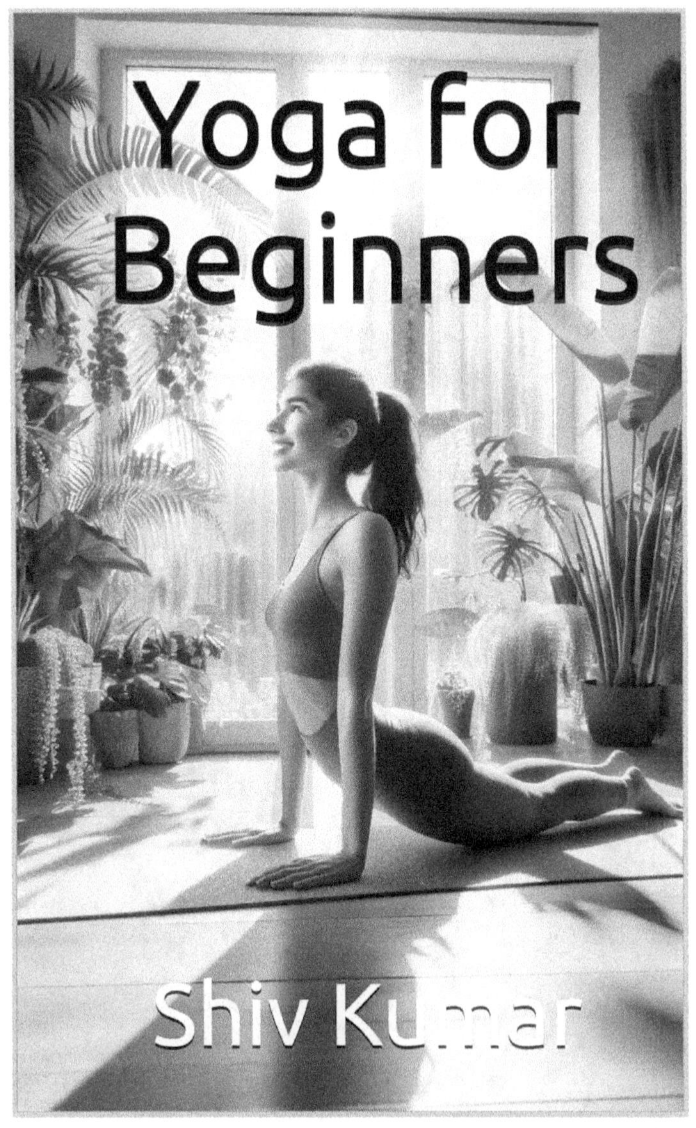
Yoga for
Beginners
Shiv Kumar